Understanding

CW00322566

SKIN
PROBLEMS

Dr Graham Colver & Dr John A. Savin

Published by Family Doctor Publications Limited
in association with the British Medical Association

IMPORTANT

This book is intended to supplement the advice given to you by your doctor. The author and publisher have taken every care in its preparation. In particular, information about drugs and dosages has been thoroughly checked. However, before taking any medication you are strongly advised to read the product information sheet accompanying it. Your pharmacist will be able to help you with anything you do not understand.

© Family Doctor Publications 1993, 1996
Reprinted 1994
Second edition 1996

Medical Editor: Dr Tony Smith
Cover Artist: Colette Blanchard
Design: MPG Design, Godalming, Surrey
Printing: Cambus Litho, Scotland, using acid-free paper

ISBN: 1 898205 06 X

Contents

Introduction

Every doctor soon learns how common and distressing skin diseases are: sufferers already know this, having found out the hard way. They account for as many as 10 per cent of all consultations in general practice; and this is only the tip of a much larger iceberg of skin disease in the community.

A study of adults in the UK, for example, found that one-quarter had a skin disorder which needed medical attention, though less than one in five of these had been shown to a doctor within the previous six months.

This is a pity and must have caused much unnecessary suffering as skin diseases can be extremely uncomfortable – indeed, itching can sometimes be worse than pain. Skin diseases can also be ugly and embarrassing.

Before discussing these problems in more detail, it is helpful to look at the structure of the skin and how it works.

THE STRUCTURE AND FUNCTION OF THE SKIN

The skin acts as a tough, self-repairing, flexible covering without which we would fall apart. It protects us from sunlight and injury. It also controls our temperature. If we get too hot we sweat and go red; the sweat evaporates and the dilated blood vessels throw off heat, and, as a result, we cool down again. The skin keeps water out and, just as important, keeps water in. If it is destroyed by an extensive burn, the uncontrolled loss of fluid will become a serious problem.

The skin consists of two layers: the epidermis and the dermis.

The epidermis

This is the layer nearest to the surface. It is about as thick as a piece of writing paper. There are no blood vessels or nerves in it, so if a pin is pushed sideways through this outer layer of skin, it will not bleed or hurt.

The skin consists essentially of two layers – dermis (true skin), which contains most of the living elements, and epidermis, which is a tough protective covering with an outer layer of dead cells.

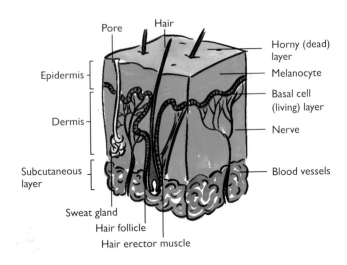

The cells in the deeper part of the epidermis divide and move outwards so that there is a continuous movement of cells towards the surface. On nearing the surface, which normally takes three to four weeks, the skin cells die and flatten out to become part of the outer, horny layer which in most areas is thin. On the palms of the hands and soles of the feet it is thicker – up to about 3 mm.

The dead cells in the horny layer are continuously shed from the surface, but in such small pieces that the skin does not normally look scaly. However, scales become obvious when the rate of shedding increases, as in psoriasis, or if the tiny fragments clump together into larger chunks as in eczema or dandruff.

The dermis

This layer lies under the epidermis and gives it support. It is made of fibres which interleave to give our skin its strength (collagen fibres) and elasticity (elastin fibres). As we age, our skin loses some of its elasticity and begins to sag and wrinkle. Any deep damage to the dermis disturbs these fibres and will leave a scar: in contrast, superficial damage to the epidermis heals quickly and without leaving any trace. Running through the dermis are blood and lymph vessels and nerves; therefore it hurts and bleeds if it is cut.

Hairs

These grow out through holes in the epidermis, but the hair follicles (roots) where they are formed lie deep in the dermis. An individual follicle goes through alternating phases of growth and rest, but not in time with its neighbours. The scalp contains about 100,000 hairs, each of which will grow for up to five years before being shed. A normal scalp can therefore lose up to 100 hairs a day just as a result of this growth/rest cycle.

Grease glands

Opening into the hair follicles are sebaceous (grease) glands which produce oil. This lubricates and waterproofs the skin, and is also mildly antiseptic. Overactive grease glands are a nuisance on the face, especially for people who suffer from acne.

Sweat glands

These are of two types. Each of us has two to three million eccrine sweat glands which produce a watery sweat – up to two to three litres a day in very hot climates. The evaporation of this helps to cool us down. It also helps with grip – it is surprisingly difficult to grip with bone-dry hands. Too much sweat may be a hindrance, but a little is necessary.

The second type of sweat gland (apocrine) is most numerous in the armpits and the groin. Skin bacteria act on their secretions to cause body odour.

COMMON CONDITIONS

The ten most common skin conditions seen in our clinics are shown below; modern treatments can now deal effectively with most of them, but left alone they can cause untold misery and even put jobs at risk.

- Virus infections (mainly warts)
- Harmless growths (e.g. skin tags, keratoses)
- Eczema
- Psoriasis
- Acne
- Fungus infections
- Skin cancer
- Urticaria
- Hair loss (alopecia)
- Moles

Eczema and dermatitis

This is a complicated subject – even the spelling of the word eczema is not easy. However, the problems have lessened now that most dermatologists agree that the words eczema and dermatitis should mean the same thing: contact eczema is therefore the same thing as contact dermatitis, atopic eczema as atopic dermatitis, etc. We take this line too, but admit that a few dermatologists still cling on to the idea that the word dermatitis applies mainly to problems of external (contact) origin.

What does eczema look like?
This depends on its type. But whatever the cause, eczema tends to go through the same stages, often showing several at the same time on different parts of the skin.

The earliest stage is for tiny, itchy blisters to appear on a red background. If the eczema is severe, or on the palms and soles, the blisters can grow quite large before they pop, and the eczema then enters the weeping stage. Later, eczema may become crusted and infected. Finally, if the condition lasts a long time, the skin will become thickened, slightly pigmented, dry and leathery with scratch marks, and an increase in the normal skin markings, but with no obvious blisters or weeping. This is chronic eczema.

The different types of eczema
Perhaps the best way of dividing eczema is into two main categories:

1. Those types caused by direct contact between the skin and an outside chemical agent (contact or exogenous eczema). Contact eczema may be due to a true allergy to the chemical in question (allergic contact eczema) or simply due to its ability to irritate the skin (irritant contact eczema).

2. Those without any obvious surface contact cause (constitutional or endogenous eczema), the most important of which are atopic, seborrhoeic and discoid eczema.

Allergic contact eczema (dermatitis)

This causes the rashes that many people get from contact with perfumes, cosmetics or jewellery. People can become allergic to things they have handled safely for years. Once allergic, they will react to the offending substance whenever and wherever it comes into contact with the skin.

Nickel is a good example, the allergy often starting after ear-piercing and then leading to rashes under cheap jewellery, jean studs, wrist watches, etc. Other common culprits include chrome in cement, sticking plaster, rubber chemicals and leather.

It may be possible to damp down reactions of this sort by using corticosteroid creams. However, a far better way of tackling the problem is first to identify the chemical in question by patch testing, and then to avoid contact with it. In nickel allergy, for example, metal bra clips can be replaced by plastic ones, pure gold and silver jewellery can replace cheaper nickel-containing items.

Patch testing is an investigation: purified chemical substances are mixed in soft paraffin and applied to the skin of the back in small chambers. If a red patch of eczema appears up to four days later it suggests that the chemical is involved somehow in the patient's eczema. One example of such a chemical is colophony (a resin used in certain chemical processes) – if it produces a red patch one would

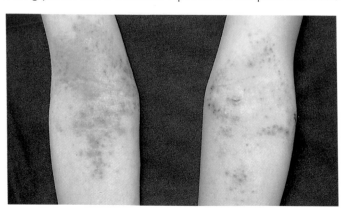

Atopic eczema.

have to think of Elastoplast, varnishes, glues, soaps and soldering agents as a cause of the eczema since they all contain colophony.

Irritant contact eczema (dermatitis)

This accounts for most industrial cases. Prolonged exposure, sometimes for years, is needed for weak irritants to cause this type of 'wear and tear' eczema. Detergents, alkalis, cutting oils and rough work are common culprits. Hairdressers, nurses, car mechanics and cleaners are at particular risk.

Skin damaged in this way, usually on the hands, may take weeks or months to return to normal, and all too often this potentially reversible condition becomes chronic. Treatment must include changes in the daily routine to reduce skin damage. Protective gloves should be worn whenever possible. At work it will be necessary to discuss the problem with the works doctor or personnel manager so that changes can be made to the current job.

Atopic eczema

This often occurs in those who have asthma or hay fever, or in their relatives. It may start at any age, but often does so in the first year of life, affecting at least one baby in 50. In infancy it may start on the face: in childhood the eczema becomes dry, leathery and heavily scratched, and lies mainly in the bends of the elbows and knees and on the wrists and ankles. Usually it clears up by the age of four or five years, but in a minority of children it may linger on beyond this age. Eczema and asthma may see-saw so that while one is improving the other may be getting worse.

The cardinal feature of atopic eczema is itching. Affected babies may rub their faces on their pillows, but as soon as their fingers can be controlled they will be used for scratching. Children with eczema may sleep poorly and be too tired to cope with their school work.

Treatment of atopic eczema

• **Emollients:** the dry, cracked skin of eczema sufferers does not tolerate soap well, and soap substitutes such as emulsifying ointment and cleansing bars are often recommended instead. Emollients are also important to replace some of the skin's natural greasiness. Sufferers vary in their preferences, but most like products which lie somewhere between light, water-based creams and greasy ointments such as Vaseline. They have to be used regularly to have any worthwhile effect.

• **Steroid creams and ointments:** these were first introduced in the 1950s and have dramatically

- Wool and many synthetic fibres can irritate the skin: pure cotton is best.
- Overheating from excessive clothing or central heating provokes itching.
- Some atopic children cannot tolerate certain foods (e.g. milk, eggs, fish). Occasionally this causes a flare-up of their eczema. More often they react by itching or swelling around the mouth or by vomiting.
- Pets may cause allergy – ideally fur and feathers should be kept out of the house.
- The evidence that early bottle feeding provokes eczema is not particularly strong, but of course there are many other good reasons for encouraging breast feeding.

improved the treatment of eczema. It is true that, if used excessively, the stronger ones may have some side effects (e.g. thinning of the skin or stretch marks), but many people have become so worried about these that they do not use enough to have any effect at all.

Hydrocortisone is both the weakest and the safest preparation, and hydrocortisone creams or ointments prescribed by a doctor may be used for children, even on their faces. In contrast, the strongest types of corticosteroid should be used only for short periods of time and never on the face.

- **Other treatments:** antibiotics may be needed if the eczema has become infected. Sedative antihistamines are of value if sleep is interrupted. In stubborn cases careful treatment with ultraviolet light may help, as may a course of evening primrose oil. Tar preparations may be applied directly to the skin or be used in impregnated bandages. Wet wraps of cotton tubular bandages may be applied over emollients – a dry cotton layer then goes over the top to contain the moisture. The role of Chinese traditional medicine is still being evaluated.

Seborrhoeic eczema

In babies this may appear as cradle cap – an accumulation of yellowish-brown scales on the scalp. Red scaly areas can also develop behind the ears and on the face, and a nappy rash may be part of the problem, too. Even then the baby remains well and happy, in contrast to the itchy, miserable one with widespread atopic eczema. The condition tends to settle slowly, over a few months, helped by hydrocortisone cream. 'Cradle cap' can be softened with olive oil so that it comes off after a few days.

Seborrhoeic eczema often affects adolescents and adults, too. Mild forms are common and include dandruff and a slight scaliness of the eyebrows or creases on either side of the nose.

More severe forms may affect the face, the centres of the back and chest, and armpits and groin. It tends to come and go: although it may occasionally be stubborn, weak steroids, antiseptics or anti-yeast preparations are usually helpful.

Discoid eczema

Round, red patches of itchy skin may occur on any part of the skin; they often weep and become covered in a yellow crust. The cause of the condition is not known, but it is seen most often in stressed, middle-aged men. Combined steroid antibiotic creams are usually needed for control, but the condition often grumbles on for many months before it goes away.

Neurodermatitis

If a patch of skin is itchy, it gets scratched. This makes it itchier than ever, so it has to be scratched again and again. Eventually the skin becomes thickened and the original cause of the itching may no longer be seen: the scratching continues as a nervous habit, which is worse when the patient is under stress. Such patches are most common on the ankles of men and at the back of the neck in women.

If the patient stops scratching, the skin will return slowly to normal, but the habit of scratching and rubbing is hard to give up. Medicated bandages may be one way to beat the scratch/itch cycle.

Pompholyx

This is a tiresome and unpleasant form of eczema. Recurrent bouts of small blisters appear, for no obvious reason, on the palms, fingers and soles. Attacks lasting a few weeks occur at irregular intervals and can be damped down with corticosteroid creams.

Stasis (varicose) eczema

This patchy, chronic eczema of the lower legs may or may not be accompanied by obvious varicose veins. Fluid and red cells leak out of the tiny vessels. The result is swelling of the ankle and a red–brown discoloration. Leg ulcers may also occur.

Ointment helps to cut down the skin dryness and steroids may have to be used on the affected area. Support stockings may also be needed, as may treatment to any varicose veins present.

Eczema of the nappy area (nappy rash)

It is unusual for any baby to cruise through the first year of its life without developing a nappy rash. This may affect all of the skin in the nappy area, or it may either favour or spare the creases. The colour may be red or pink and the skin may be scaly and thickened, thin and shiny, or even covered in small ulcers.

The common causes are irritation from a soiled nappy, seborrhoeic eczema or infection with yeasts. Often, several of these factors act together so that an area of mild seborrhoeic eczema may quickly become painful and soggy after contact with stale urine. Friction will also aggravate any type of nappy rash.

Treatment should begin with general measures. The baby's bottom should be kept clean by gentle wiping with cotton wool moistened with mild, unperfumed soap and water or an oily cream. The skin should then be patted dry. The nappy should be changed frequently (immediately if it is soiled) and nappy liners should be used with terry napkins. Thorough rinsing of washed towelling nappies is also important. Ointment (e.g. zinc and castor oil), which can be bought from the chemist, may be used to protect the damaged skin.

FURTHER POINTS

Eczema affects people differently. The most obvious changes are in the skin, but many other aspects of life are changed too, for example, self-esteem, relationships with other people and sex life. Time may have to be taken off work for medical attendances. Your doctor is likely to have come across all these problems before. Do ask about what is on your mind.

The National Eczema Society (see page 58) is also there to give advice and has the experience of thousands of eczema subjects on which to call. It produces helpful leaflets on all aspects of the condition. Write for further information, enclosing a stamped, self-addressed envelope.

Psoriasis

In Britain about one person in 50 has psoriasis. People are often surprised by this, and wonder why they do not come across it more often. The reason is that most sufferers have little to show for much of the time – what psoriasis they have is often just on the elbows and knees and covered by clothes.

In addition, there is often a marked improvement in the summer months so that, in some, the scaly skin disappears entirely, while in others it may only be minimal. Certainly a lot of psoriasis sufferers look forward to the summer and others take an early foreign break in the spring to try and get their skin clear.

Why do some people get psoriasis?

Psoriasis does run in families – if one of your parents has the disease, your own chance of getting it at some stage is about one in four. But even in identical twins there may be only one who is affected; there are many people with psoriasis who cannot trace anyone in the family who has had it. Psoriasis is clearly not inherited in any simple way.

Many doctors now believe that what is passed down is a tendency to get psoriasis, but it has to be brought out by something else such as a bad throat infection, other infections, medication or severe stress. Some people carrying this tendency to get psoriasis go through life without the disease ever being triggered off at all, but they may still pass the tendency on to their own children.

What does psoriasis look like?

Psoriasis can be identified readily enough. Its pink/red patches are covered in whitish scales. In black people the patches are rather darker than the surrounding skin and the red element is less obvious. The edges of each patch are clear cut and do not fade out gradually like eczema. If scaling is heavy, whiteness becomes the most obvious feature. However, when the scale is rubbed off, the red/pink colour appears. These patches can vary in size from a pinhead to a dinner plate, but most are an inch or two across.

Psoriasis does not obey any rules. Any part of the body may be affected, but especially the points of the elbows and knees and the scalp. Scars often become involved by psoriasis and this is called the Koebner phenomenon. Luckily, it does not usually affect the face.

SPECIAL PATTERNS OF PSORIASIS

Plaque psoriasis
This type is slow to come and slow to go; the areas commonly affected are the elbows and knees and the lower back. Cracks appear if the skin becomes too dry and are painful, especially over a joint during movement. Very scaly plaques can shed showers of embarrassing scales.

Some people become extremely concerned about leaving behind a trail of scales. They go as far as not visiting other people's houses and, if they stay at an hotel, taking a mini-vacuum to clear up the mess.

Guttate psoriasis
Hundreds of little areas, like drops of water, develop rapidly, especially on the trunk. This type may erupt a week or so after a throat infection, and is common in young people. If it repeatedly follows tonsillitis, removal of the tonsils may be recommended. Guttate psoriasis often improves by itself over a couple of months, but it can also be helped to clear by creams and ultraviolet light.

Flexural psoriasis
This is psoriasis in the skin creases, e.g. armpits, under the breasts, between the buttocks and in the groin. It may occur with other types of psoriasis, but it looks different –

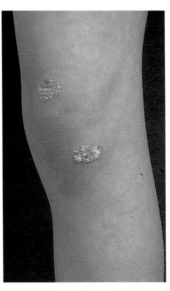

Mild psoriasis.

there is no scale and the skin appears red and shiny.

Pustular psoriasis

In this type, groups of tiny yellow blisters form. They are not caused by infection, but by an active form of the disease which attracts many white blood cells to the area. One chronic type of pustular psoriasis, on the palms and soles, is particularly difficult to treat. A more worrying variation is the appearance of pustules, anywhere on the skin, during an exacerbation of the disease. The eruptions become unstable and treatment must be carefully supervised, often in hospital.

Scalp and nails

Occasionally these may be the only areas affected, but more often the changes accompany disease elsewhere on the body.

The scalp may become scaly at the edges or all over, and build up quickly to form a thick layer that is difficult to treat. Nails can be a major problem; although a minor pitting and roughening is often seen, the whole nail may occasionally become grossly thickened, awkward to use and unattractive. Another change is a lifting-off of the nail plate from the underlying bed, allowing air and dirt to enter and causing discomfort and disfigurement.

Erythroderma

This literally means a red skin. On rare occasions psoriasis gets out of control and the plaques lose their normal appearance. Hugh areas of skin can then become hot, red and dry. If this happens consult a doctor who may suggest that you should spend time in hospital

Acrostic

It is difficult to sum up all the adverse effects of psoriasis. One sufferer, an eloquent graphic designer, summed up his psoriasis thus.

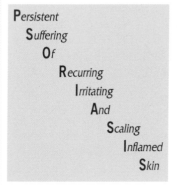

Persistent
Suffering
Of
Recurring
Irritating
And
Scaling
Inflamed
Skin

TREATMENT

Most people with psoriasis will tell you that, at times, their skin gets better for no obvious reason. As with many illnesses, if life becomes chaotic and stressful, the symptoms get worse. Psoriasis may therefore break out in stressful conditions, but stress is not its sole cause.

Diet

Diets are fashionable and, with herbal remedies, make up a huge business. They have always been popular and new ideas are always being put forward. Fish oil is an example of a recent fad. Overall, however, doctors are not impressed by the value of special diets; at best they usually only have a tiny part to play.

Holidays

Holidays are good for psoriasis. Sunlight has a special value and will be discussed later, but relaxation is also beneficial.

Moisturisers

Greasy skin preparations help as psoriasis tends to be dry. Anything from white soft paraffin to a light hand cream will help, and people vary in their individual preferences. They may ease dryness and actually help to heal the disease.

Coal tar

Tars are among the oldest remedies. They are made by the distillation of wood or coal, and the exact constituents depend on the raw materials. There are literally thousands of chemicals in tar, only a few of which have been identified. Pharmaceutical companies have produced a range of preparations based on tar. Some are smelly, staining and thick. Others are clean, odourless and creamy. Unfortunately the nicest creams tend to be the least effective. In addition, some people find that tar irritates their skin, but this is usually a temporary problem.

Dithranol

This can be very helpful and works by slowing down the rate at which skin cells divide. Originally derived from trees, dithranol can now be synthesised in the laboratory. At one time its use was largely restricted to patients in hospital, but some of its problems have been resolved by modern preparations.

It is available in creams and ointments, and in various strengths. It should be applied to only the affected skin, and can be left on all day but leaves a brown stain on surrounding skin, clothes, fingers, hair and bedclothes. Every week or so the strength can be increased, but if the skin becomes sore the treatment should be left off for a few days.

Recently, higher concentrations of dithranol (in a vanishing cream base) have been used in the short contact method. The cream is left on the skin for 30 minutes, then washed off. This is just as effective as the old method, but does not spoil clothes or bedclothes.

Calcipotriol

This exciting compound is derived

WHAT IT MEANS TO HAVE PSORIASIS

- **Soreness** when cracks appear over joints.
- **Itching:** not common, but troubles some people a lot.
- **Scales** may look like dandruff and flake on the floor.
- **Ability to carry out day-to-day tasks** may be affected. There are many examples of this: affected feet may limit walking, nails may interfere with picking items up and plaques on the knees make kneeling awkward.
- **Disfigurement:** psoriasis affects self-esteem if the red, scaly patches are visible. Sufferers may be too embarrassed to go swimming, sunbathe or to let friends see their skin. Unfortunately some unaffected people have an irrational fear of diseased skin which makes them do and say silly, hurtful things. Psoriasis is not infectious, but in a swimming pool people may seem to be keeping well away from the sufferer.
- **Employment:** functional impairment may affect employment and those who spend a lot of time at or in hospital may find that their employers object.

from vitamin D and is now available as a safe and cosmetically acceptable ointment. In Britain it is marketed as Dovonex. Although it does not suit everyone, there is no doubt that it has made a big difference to many psoriasis sufferers.

Steroid creams

Mild steroid creams, such as hydrocortisone, have little effect on psoriasis except in the skin creases and on the face. Stronger steroids can be dramatically effective, particularly in the first few weeks of use. However, most doctors feel that their use should be restricted to a few weeks and to certain situations. These include sore or inflamed psoriasis, pustular disease of the palms and soles, and when there is a need for rapid clearance, e.g. before a wedding. If steroids are used excessively there is a danger of thinning the skin, and if they are withdrawn suddenly there is a risk of the psoriasis deteriorating rapidly.

Ultraviolet

Ultraviolet light itself is not visible, but usually the lamps which produce it also give out some visible light. There are three wavebands of ultraviolet light called UV-A, UV-B and UV-C. The band most commonly used in treatment is UV-B, which can be given by a single lamp or in a chamber whose walls are lined by many fluorescent tubes. Treatment is given two or three times a week in increasing doses. It is not necessary to turn red to derive benefit and, indeed, a burn can be counterproductive.

UV-A is normally given with psoralen tablets, and the combination is called PUVA. The drug sensitises the skin and is given an hour before UV-A exposure. The whole body is treated in a cabinet twice a week.

Most sunlamps for home use are obviously designed for safety. Manufacturers are keen to avoid burning their clients. Much of the irradiation is UV-A, which burns less than UV-B. Infrared light is also given off, but this simply warms and soothes the body.

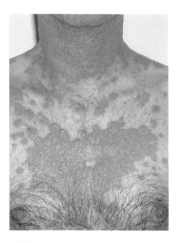
Widespread thin patches of psoriasis.

Special dark glasses must be worn when the body is exposed to any form of ultraviolet light, and, after PUVA, they should be kept on until nightfall.

Powerful drugs

For many years methotrexate has been of value in treating people with severe psoriasis resistant to standard methods. It is a drug used also in cancer therapy because of its ability to stop the division of certain cells. In psoriasis it has this beneficial effect on skin cells, but also has unwanted actions on the bone marrow and liver. Careful monitoring of regular blood tests is therefore needed.

Another drug is acitretin, derived from vitamin A. It reduces the thickness of plaques and improves the pustular forms of psoriasis. Side effects include a rise in blood cholesterol, redness and dry lips, but, most importantly, damage to an unborn child. The fetus can be seriously affected if the mother takes the drug during pregnancy or even if she stopped taking it a year or two beforehand.

Cyclosporin A is another new drug with a place in the treatment of severe psoriasis, but, again, there are many potential problems and its use is restricted.

Psoriatic arthritis

About one person in 20 with

psoriasis develops some joint troubles, though these are usually mild. Finger and toe joints are the most common sites, and often there are pits or other changes in the nails of the affected digits.

Almost any joint may be a problem in psoriasis, but of course arthritis and psoriasis are common diseases and the two may exist together by chance in some people.

SUPPORT

The Psoriasis Association (see page 58) is run for people with psoriasis by people with psoriasis. They will always give you sound advice about different treatments, information about living with the disease and the benefit of the experience that other members have had with both conventional and unconventional treatments.

Acne

Acne is something everyone can recognise easily enough. If you look closely, however, you can see that it is made up of a mixture of different types of spot, usually against a rather greasy background skin. There are inflamed spots (papules), some of which turn into yellow heads containing pus; blackheads or comedones (pronounced commy-doans) can also occur in profusion; deep and tender lumps are known as nodules and cysts; finally, the scars which affect a minority of people are permanent and should, therefore, be prevented from forming if possible. All of these blemishes are based on hair follicles.

Acne usually starts at puberty and only three out of ten teenagers escape unscathed. It affects so many people that it can even be regarded as a normal part of growing up. Nevertheless, though it is mild in some, it is painful and severe in others and the ways in which skins respond to treatment also vary enormously. During the past ten years there have been great gains in our understanding of acne and in the treatment of its more severe forms. Mild acne has been satisfactorily treated for several years.

WHAT CAUSES ACNE?

The heart of the problem, in acne, lies in the sebaceous (grease) glands. These are found all over the skin, except on the palms and soles, but are most numerous on the face where there are about 600 to a square centimetre. They produce a greasy fluid called sebum, and in adolescence enlarge and produce more sebum in response to rising hormone levels. The important hormone controlling the grease glands is the male sex hormone testosterone. Low levels are found in all women, but it is this small amount which gives rise to acne. Castrated men (eunuchs) have virtually no testosterone and do not get acne – an interesting but unhelpful fact.

Increased sebum does not cause acne by itself. The openings through which hairs leave the skin are called pilosebaceous orifices or pores. They are so tiny that any disturbance of the surrounding skin

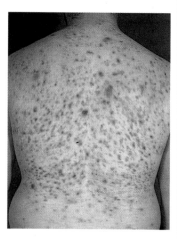

Extensive acne on the back.

will lead to a blockage. Increased hormone levels created just this situation: the superficial cells do not brush off the surface normally but tend to stick together and block the pores. Sebum is immediately dammed back, and this combination of events produces blackheads. The retained sebum acts as an excellent growth medium for certain skin bacteria.

Proprionibacterium acnes

These bacteria are normally harmless, but in increased numbers can change the constituents of the sebum so that it irritates the surrounding skin. They also attract white blood cells which produce inflammation, papules and subsequently pustules. If the glands swell greatly, cysts may be formed and cause discomfort.

THINGS THAT HELP – AND SOME THAT DON'T

Often old wives' tales hold more than a grain of truth, but in acne, most of the widely held beliefs are wrong. Does diet, in particular greasy food or chocolate, affect acne? The answer seems to be 'no'.

Nevertheless, some people insist that a certain food makes their acne worse, in which case it seems sensible to avoid it. Years ago, in America, a group of young prisoners was fed huge quantities of chocolate daily for several weeks. They had no more acne at the end of the experiment than a similar group of prisoners on a normal diet.

Fresh air and exercise

People often ask whether exercise and outdoor activities help acne. Sunlight may, and indeed it is often used in treatment. However, any other improvements are due more to the confidence given by such pursuits than to any changes in the skin. Sexual activity, or lack of it, does not alter acne in any way.

Occupation and environment

It is more common for acne to interfere with employment than vice versa. For example, acne sufferers are often embarrassed in jobs with much public exposure. Sometimes an employer may think that it will affect business to have an employee with a spotty face dealing with clients. Jobs in hot climates can be a real problem. Acne may worsen in moist tropical climates, especially if washing facilities are poor.

Similar conditions prevail in certain occupations, e.g. bakers, boilermakers, fish and chip shop workers, and actors. A more serious occupational acne is seen in people exposed to certain chlorine-containing chemicals. Such contact may be brief or accidental, after a leak or explosion, but the effects can be severe.

The last type to mention here is acne brought on, or worsened, by medicinal drugs. One example of this is epilepsy treatment (anti-convulsants) and other high-dose steroids, which occasionally produce an acute papular and pustular eruption on the upper trunk and face.

Hormones

Girls and young women often find that acne gets worse around the time of their period. This effect is hormone related, but varies from person to person. The contraceptive pill may help some people and this is discussed under medical treatment.

Herbal remedies

These are difficult to assess because their manufacturers never compare them with other treatments. Herbalists use vague terms like 'detoxifying the tissues' and 'purifying the blood'. They also focus on dietary measures. Surely, if any method had been consistently effective we should all know about it by now.

Squeezing spots

Do not pick or squeeze your spots as this can lead to more inflammation and scars. Once there was a fashion for dealing with blackheads using special extractors, but these are generally not recommended now. When a blackhead is ready to come away it takes only a little persuasion; when it is not, fiddling with it is rather like trying to get an unripe conker out of its shell – it damages the skin.

Washing and cosmetics

Very greasy or oily cosmetics are best avoided because they can block up the follicles and make matters worse. This may happen under a fringe when the hair prevents grease from escaping. In Britain most doctors are happy to allow the use of non-comedogenic foundation, moisturisers, etc. Washing of the skin should be with normal soap or cleansing bars. Strangely, it seems that some people who become obsessional face-washers, washing about six times a day, can also develop acne for the first time.

MEDICAL TREATMENT

This may be a long process. Of course, very mild acne responds rapidly to therapy, which may involve the use of a single cream. However, most forms, and particularly severe acne, take weeks or months to improve. Sometimes there may be no visible gain for two months, and it is easy to become disheartened.

Sulphur and antiseptics

Sulphur was once popular, but it is seldom used today. It smells unpleasant and encourages the formation of blackheads. Antiseptics are of some value, and are sold in large quantities across the counter. The single most popular agent now used by doctors is benzoyl peroxide, which has been around for at least 20 years. It acts as an antiseptic, killing bacteria, but it also reduces sebum excretion and loosens blackheads so that they come away more readily. It comes in strengths of 2.5, 5 and 10 per cent, and in a variety of creams, lotions and gels. Benzoyl peroxide often irritates the skin so that people discard it without more ado. Redness and scaling are common in the first few weeks of use, but the skin must be coaxed into accepting it. Start by leaving it on for only a few hours and then washing it off. If the skin becomes sore stop for three or four days and then try again. Most people start with 5 per cent and may later move on to the 10 per cent preparation.

Skin on the face is more sensitive than that on the chest or back, and may need the lower concentration. Remember that, even though it takes weeks to work, benzoyl peroxide provides an enormous benefit for mild to moderate acne. Some sufferers can control their acne with it alone over many years.

Creams related to vitamin A

Retin A and Isotrex are two commercial preparations derived from this natural vitamin. Vitamin A is known to have a controlling effect on the development of normal skin so it is not surprising that these creams can reduce both sebum production and the number of blackheads. Their role in wrinkle therapy is more controversial.

Ultraviolet light

Sunlight improves the skin of most acne sufferers. It is particularly useful for the smaller red spots and blackheads. At one time it was a common treatment in hospital, but modern creams are usually every bit as good.

Antibiotics

If other approaches are not successful, or if the acne is particularly bad, antibiotic tablets are normally given. The main ones are tetracycline and erythromycin. They kill bacteria but also seem to reduce inflammation. Always follow the instructions on how and when to take them; oxytetracycline in particular is poorly absorbed from a stomach which has food in it. Headaches and queasiness are quite common while taking these drugs.

As with other therapies for acne, the benefits take a while to appear and at least four months' treatment is the rule.

Hormone therapy

The contraceptive pill Dianette is discussed fully in the chapter on excess hair growth. It works in a similar manner in acne, but can, of course, only be used in women. Again, it takes months to have much effect.

Roaccutane

Roaccutane was introduced about 15 years ago and is having a dramatic effect on the treatment of severe acne. There are side effects such as dry, red, scaly skin, cracked lips, sore muscles and minor nose bleeds. Occasionally it temporarily elevates the blood cholesterol level. If pregnancy occurs while taking the drug, or soon afterwards, it can even cause severe fetal abnormalities. However, this drug has revolutionised the lives of many acne sufferers and should always be considered if acne is have a profound effect on life. Roaccutane can only be prescribed in hospitals.

OUTLOOK

Acne is active in many people, to some degree, from the age of 12 to about 24. At different stages it may need only creams or creams plus tablets.

Unfortunately there are still a few youngsters who have severe acne which does not respond fully to therapy, but on the whole there is now an excellent and ever improving range of acceptable medications to cope with all degrees of this common and disfiguring disease.

Urticaria

Urticaria (nettle rash or hives) is a rash made up of itchy weals. At the onset these are raised and red, but later they become white in the centre with a red rim around. Weals vary in size from small ones like a nettle sting to much large ones several centimetres across. An individual weal may only last up to 48 hours, but while one is clearing, another may be forming so that the process goes on for several weeks or months.

What is the cause of urticaria?

The weals come up in response to the release in the skin of a chemical known as histamine. This makes small skin blood vessels so permeable that they leak fluid into the surrounding tissues causing visible swelling.

The most difficult problem with urticaria is to find what is causing the histamine to be released in the first place. Short-lived attacks of urticaria may follow an obvious allergy, for example, to a penicillin injection or to eating shellfish. All too often, however, patients continue to have urticaria for longer periods and then the cause is seldom found. Even allergy testing is not helpful.

Sometimes the cause of the urticaria is an extreme sensitivity of the skin to minor pressure; the weals then tend to look long and thin, rather than round, as they follow the lines where the fingers have scratched the skin.

How can urticaria be treated?

Antihistamine medicines, given by mouth, are the mainstay of treatment in urticaria. They block the actions of histamine on the skin and so suppress the uncomfortable rash, but they do not stop histamine being released so the weals will often come back if treatment is stopped.

In some cases other chemicals are released in the skin too, so that antihistamines may not be completely effective. Some antihistamines make people drowsy, and mix badly with alcohol or sleeping pills. Care may be needed when driving a car or working with machinery. Many of the newer antihistamines do not have this sedative effect.

Patients with urticaria should avoid medicines containing aspirin and its derivatives as these may help to liberate more histamine. Exclusive diets that contain no food additives have also been tried with mixed success.

Infections

When people talk about germs they really mean bacteria, viruses or fungi. These are all microscopic organisms that can either exist harmlessly on the skin or cause diseases.

Resistance to them varies. Some people seem to have naturally poor resistance and are always picking up colds or repeated boils.

Environmental factors include heat because many organisms thrive in the warmth. Sunlight itself can induce a viral cold sore.

Many infections can pass from person to person so it makes sense to avoid direct contact if possible. For example, someone with an active cold sore should avoid kissing anyone and a child with untreated impetigo (see page 25) should be kept away from other children.

BACTERIAL INFECTIONS

Folliculitis

This is a mild infection of the hair follicles caused by bacteria called staphylococci. Pus spots appear in hairy areas such as the upper thighs, being commoner in hot climates and under tight fitting clothes. Treatment includes avoidance of these causes and applying antiseptic creams. Antibiotics are not usually required.

Boils and carbuncles

These are deeper infections of hair follicles, but the same bacteria are to blame. With a boil, a painful red lump enlarges, points and eventually bursts, letting out yellow pus.

A carbuncle involves several hair follicles close together, and forms an even larger swelling which may ooze pus through many openings. Early treatment with an antibiotic by mouth is advisable, but later it may be necessary to open a boil with a scalpel.

Anyone who develops repeated boils should consult their doctor so that diseases which reduce immunity, e.g. diabetes, can be eliminated. In addition they may be harbouring the germs in their noses and will need to apply antibiotic ointment there regularly. Family members should be treated in the same way in case one of them is carrying the germs without having boils themselves.

Impetigo

This may be due to staphylococci, streptococci or both. Spots commonly start around the mouth, nose, ears or armpits as thin-walled blisters filled with runny pus. These rupture leaving a golden crust under which lies a red, weeping area. Scratching helps to spread impetigo around the body, and it passes readily to other people.

Early cases can be treated with warm olive oil to remove the crusts and then by antibiotic cream. People with bad attacks need an antibiotic by mouth, too, and affected children should be kept off school and use a separate flannel and towel until the disease has settled.

Erysipelas

The bacterium to blame for this infection is another streptococcus. It gets into the skin through tiny cracks and favours areas such as the webs of fingers and under the earlobes. Pus does not form, but the infection spreads quickly as a red, hot, swollen area. At an early stage the patient feels shivery and ill and needs urgent treatment with an appropriate antibiotic. Penicillin is often the best.

Cellulitis

In many ways this is similar to erysipelas, but the bacteria are different and the infection is deeper in the tissues. It may appear around surgical wounds and leg ulcers. One part of the body may be attacked repeatedly over many years and permanent swelling may follow.

VIRAL INFECTIONS

Viruses are smaller than bacteria and can only be seen with an electron microscope. Everyone is aware of viruses that cause diseases associated with a rash, for example, measles. In this chapter we deal only with those that give problems predominantly on the skin.

Warts

These are a common nuisance. It is now known that several strains of wart virus exist, each tending to cause its own type of wart, such as

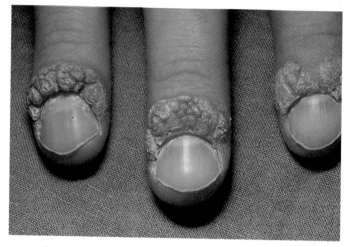

Large and thick warts around the nail folds. These are hard to treat.

common warts on the hand, painful ones on the feet (verucca), facial warts and genital warts.

Although each type needs its own treatment, most will go away by themselves but may take a year or two to do so. About 35 per cent of patients lose their warts within six months, 50 per cent within one year and 67 per cent within two years. When warts go of their own accord they leave no scar or mark behind. Any treatment which leaves scars is therefore worse than doing nothing at all.

Warts are caught from other people. This happens easily in children who have not developed immunity, but with some difficulty in adults. The virus may lie dormant in the skin for months before warts appear.

Treatment depends on the age of the patient and on the type of wart. Painful methods are best avoided in children – perhaps their warts might clear up more speedily, but children can quickly become frightened of doctors and are hard to examine when more important illnesses crop up later. Wart paints are often effective and can be applied daily by parents without any fuss.

The wart should be rubbed with a pumice or emery board first. Most warts will then disappear in a few weeks. If not, in older patients they can be frozen with a very cold liquid (usually liquid nitrogen) which can be sprayed or dabbed on with a cotton-wool bud.

A verucca may be painful to walk on; rubbing it down with a

pumice stone may then be all that is required. Veruccas should only be treated if they are troublesome. However, you should cover them if you have a communal shower after sports. Soggy feet are always likely to pick up the virus, so plastic socks are supplied at swimming pools.

Genital warts require different treatment and this should include an examination of sexual partners as well as a search for other sexually acquired diseases. Various methods of treatment are available, but all must be used regularly; even so, relapses are quite common.

Molluscum contagiosum

This common viral infection is often referred to as 'water warts'. It mainly affects children and particularly those who suffer from eczema. Its tiny spots look rather like drops of milk, but through a lens each can be seen to have a little dimple in its centre. The virus can be spread around the body by scratching. Most new mollusca appear in groups near existing ones, but a few may crop up at a distance.

Molluscum can also spread from person to person – hence the word

HERPES SIMPLEX

The primary infection normally occurs in childhood as a blistering rash on the lips and mouth in an unwell child. The virus is never properly eliminated from the body and tends to keep coming back in roughly the same place. Cold sores are most common on the lips and around the nose and mouth. Attacks may be triggered by feverish colds, sunlight, menstruation or even stress. Tingling and burning feelings are followed within a few hours by redness on top of which are clusters of small, tense blisters. The area becomes crusty within a day or so, and clears up in about a week. Healing can sometimes be speeded up by an antiviral paint or cream, applied frequently during the first day or two of an attack. An oral treatment (acyclovir) is even more effective, but it is extremely expensive and better reserved for more serious herpes infections. A more recent drug (famciclovir) may be better still in some severe cases. The commonest way of catching herpes is by close physical contact – if you have a cold sore it is up to you not to spread it to others. Children with atopic eczema are particularly vulnerable to this virus, and can have very severe attacks; they must be protected from the virus.

contagiosum. Commonsense precautions to prevent its spread within the family include stopping children from sharing baths and towels.

The spots of molluscum do go away by themselves, but may take many months to do so. They can be hurried up in adults by various means.

These include gentle squeezing with fine forceps, freezing with liquid nitrogen, applying a wart paint or spiking with a sharpened orange stick that has been dipped into 40 per cent trichloroacetic acid. These methods are too painful for small children with many spots. An alternative is to soak in a bath for 10 minutes, then, holding the skin on either side firmly, to rub the molluscum with a pumice stone.

Unfortunately, even when all the visible lesions have been treated, more may appear as the skin has already been inoculated with a virus which continues to multiply and grow.

Herpes zoster (shingles)

Shingles is seen most often in older people. An attack frequently begins with pain but no rash. At this stage it can be hard to diagnose and the pain may be mistaken for lumbago or appendicitis. Painful blisters then appear and may be blood-filled. The blisters often form a band around part of the trunk or a line down part of a limb. The discomfort may be mild but is more often unpleasant. Near the eye there can be serious consequences. Following an acute attack, pain may continue for months or years – it is unpleasant and, when persistent, leads to depression. The same virus causes chickenpox and it is possible to catch chickenpox from someone who has got shingles.

INFECTIONS CAUSED BY YEASTS AND FUNGI

Ringworm

Several different fungi can infect the skin, hair and nails. Those that have become adapted to life on humans cause little inflammation – for example, athletes' foot may consist only of soggy areas between the toes. Fungi that normally live on animals, e.g. cattle and mouse ringworm, cause more inflammation. Hot climates, sweating and close fitting clothes all help the fungus to thrive, leading to

HAND, FOOT AND MOUTH DISEASE

This gives rise to small blisters on the hands, feet and lining of the mouth, but there are rarely many other symptoms and treatment is not usually required.

especially extensive infections.

On the trunk ringworm appears as red, itchy and scaly areas with an advancing border. The centre heals, leaving a scaly circle, hence the name. The most common sites are the groins, buttocks and armpits. On the palms and soles a chronic scaling may be seen, looking rather like dermatitis. One or more nails can be affected, showing either a white, smooth surface, a yellow crumbling or even gross destruction of the whole nail. On the scalp there may be scaling with hair loss, but little inflammation, although other fungi cause swelling, pain and pus formation around the hair follicles.

Before treatment it is important to make a firm diagnosis. Specimens of skin scale, broken off hair shafts or nail clippings can be examined under the microscope and sent to a laboratory for culture and identification. Some fungi on the scalp fluoresce under ultraviolet light. Most infections of the skin settle with antifungal creams used for a few weeks. Underlying problems should also be tackled – athletes' foot is common in miners and remains difficult to clear while they work in a warm, moist environment. Infections of hair and nails need treatment by mouth. For many years griseofulvin was the only drug available, but alternatives have appeared recently. Terbinafine

CANDIDA

This yeast is responsible for the disease known as thrush, which is common in the mouth and vagina, and on the penis. It may also occur in the groin, round the anus and, in babies, over the entire nappy area. The skin looks bright and even shiny. Outside the main area tiny satellite spots or pustules can be seen.

Effective therapy must include weight reduction and the avoidance of tight clothes and a humid environment. Antifungal creams work here also, but it may be necessary to take oral drugs in some cases, e.g. fluconazole (Diflucan). When immunity is reduced, candida tends to appear and can be very troublesome. This is the case in many people with AIDS or diabetes.

(Lamisil) and itraconazole (Sporanox) deal effectively with even severe infections and involved nails. They need only be taken for a short time to achieve success. All take a while to act and nail infections carry a small risk of recurrence once the tablets have been stopped.

Tinea versicolor

This yeast infection is more common in hot countries. It appears on the back, chest, upper arms and neck as small, slightly scaly patches. Their colour is variable, ranging from white through pink to an orangey brown. They are often noticed after a sunny holiday, partly because the skin has been exposed to view and also because the affected areas do not take a suntan, and by remaining pale become highlighted.

The condition can be diagnosed easily by looking at scrapings down the microscope. The yeast clears quickly after the application of selenium sulphide shampoo or suitable creams. However, in some resistant cases it is necessary to take a short course of itraconazole. Normal pigmentation does not return for some months and such slow improvement often leads people to believe that the treatment has failed.

INFESTATIONS

These are caused by tiny parasites that are usually just visible to the naked eye. Infestations that involve the skin, e.g. scabies and lice, are common and cause much discomfort.

Scabies

Scabies is an infestation with a tiny mite, *Sarcoptes scabei*, less than one-twentieth of an inch long. The mite is passed from person to person by close contact – it cannot

THREE TYPES OF LICE

- **Head lice:** these are common in children. Their eggs, called nits, are oval and shiny and are easily seen stuck onto the hair shafts. The skin changes are variable, but usually include redness and scratch marks as well as the nits. Spread is by close contact, especially when children play together. It has nothing to do with poor hygiene. The nits remain alive on brushed-out hairs, so the practice of sharing combs is best avoided.

- **Body lice:** these are seldom seen today. There is widespread itching and pigmentation is seen over much of the body. The lice feed on the skin, but live and lay their eggs in the seams of items of clothing.

- **Pubic lice:** crab lice infest the pubic hair and occasionally other hairy areas of the body. Patients usually make their own diagnosis after they have been itching for a while. Intimate contact is the usual method of spread, but shared towels and clothing are another source of infestation.

jump. It rapidly spreads between bedfellows but less easily through simple, everyday contact. Holding hands for a while, or a child sitting on an adult's knee, can be enough to allow it to spread. The mite cannot survive for long on clothing or sheets. Female mites burrow just under the skin surface where they lay eggs.

For the first month or so there may be little or no itching, but then the irritation becomes severe and dominates the picture, particularly at night.

There are small, red spots, dry patches and sometimes definite short, scaly burrows. The soft skin around the finger webs, wrists, waist, armpits and nipples tends to be the worst affected. The whole skin becomes itchy with the exception of the head and neck.

Treatment works well, but the lotion or cream (of which there are several good brands, e.g. Quellada and Lyclear) must be applied to the whole skin surface from the neck down. It should be washed off after 12 hours. It is important to consult your doctor before treating young children.

The whole family and close contacts should be treated, whether or not they are itchy, since some may be in the incubation stage. After successful treatment several weeks may pass before the itching settles completely.

Lice

Three types of louse affect humans – head, body and pubic lice. All feed exclusively on blood by puncturing the skin. Their saliva contains an anticoagulant. The puncture marks irritate and often become infected.

Gamma-benzene hexachloride and malathion are effective treatments for lice. A fine-tooth comb helps to remove nits from the scalp. It is wise to repeat treatments weekly for a couple of weeks in case further eggs hatch out. Family members and class mates should all be carefully checked.

PAPULAR URTICARIA

This is a common condition, particularly in children. Groups of raised, itchy spots or blisters arise on the legs and trunk. Itching is so intense that the tops are quickly scratched off the spots, causing scars which may become infected. The spots are due to insect bites, but it may not always be possible to identify the insect in question. Dog and cat fleas are commonly to blame, but most pets carry mites which may be responsible. Brushings from bedding and clothing can be examined micro-scopically. Fortunately the strong skin reaction that produces papular urticaria always settles down in the end, but may take months to do so.

Skin tumours

The word tumour often causes unnecessary alarm. It means nothing more than a swelling or a lump raised above the skin surface. It is true that some tumours are cancerous, but most are not. The word can even be applied to something as harmless and benign as an ordinary wart.

HARMLESS SKIN TUMOURS
Cysts

Several types of cyst can occur in the skin. The most common are usually still called sebaceous cysts, though strictly speaking they have no connection with the sebaceous (grease) glands. They are found most often on the scalp and run in some families. They are easy to recognise being raised, skin coloured and dome-like: some show an obvious blocked pore. The main problems are their ugly appearance and a tendency to become infected.

These cysts consists of a cheesy material lying inside a sac. Treatment is simple if the cyst has never been infected – the sac can easily be freed and pulled out intact through a slit in the skin. Unfortunately, in some cases, past infection has the effect of sticking the sac down and making removal more difficult.

Seborrhoeic warts (keratoses)

These common and harmless skin growths have a rough or warty surface, and range from light brown to black in colour. Some people have several and they tend to increase in number with age, growing mainly on the trunk and temples.

Doctors can identify most seborrhoeic warts easily enough, but occasionally this is more difficult and the wart then has to be removed and checked in detail under the microscope.

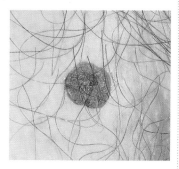

Typical seborrhoeic wart.

Seborrhoeic warts remain benign and can safely be left alone. Ugly or inconvenient ones can be destroyed by freezing with liquid nitrogen or scraped off under local anaesthetic.

Skin tags

These are little pear-shaped pieces of skin that grow out from the neck, armpits or groins and look like a crop of tiny squashed mushrooms. They are most common in middle and old age and in fat people. If they are troublesome it is easy enough for a doctor to snip them off. A popular alternative is to tie a piece of thread around the stalk and the tag will then drop off in its own time.

Keloids

The most obvious response to an injury is a scar. If this becomes lumpy, painful or itchy and larger than the original wound it is called a keloid. Lumpy scars and keloids are most likely to crop up on the skin between the nipples and the nose and some races, for example, Afro-Caribbeans, suffer particularly from this problem.

Surgeons never want to cut out keloids because another one is likely to form around the new wound. Keloids can, however, be helped by the injection of steroids and also tend slowly to improve with time.

Pyogenic granulomas

They are tiresomely named, red, raised, sometimes raspberry-like growths that come up often in children or young adults, sometimes after a prick from a sharp object. They bleed easily and are a nuisance; they should always be seen by a doctor, although they are benign. Removal of pyogenic granulomas is simple and worthwhile.

Dermatofibromas

These are firm but benign nodules usually less than 1 cm across, which are found most commonly on the arms and legs of women. They show an iceberg effect in that they feel larger than they look. They are often lightly pigmented and dimple when squeezed.

Some seem to follow minor injuries or insect bites. They can easily be removed, but often the scar left by doing this is as ugly as the original fibroma itself.

Lipomas

These are common benign tumours made up of fat. They have an irregular lobulated shape and a curious rubbery feel, and lie just under the skin. They may be multiple and are most often found on the limbs. They need to be removed only if there is doubt about the diagnosis or if they are painful or ugly.

Corns and callosities

Both of these are responses of the skin to pressure. A callosity is a diffuse thickening of the outer (keratin) layer which seems to be a protective response to widely applied, repeated friction or pressure. Callosities may be work related; they are often seen on the hands of manual workers. They are usually painless and need no treatment.

Corns have a central core of hard keratin which can hurt if forced inwards. They come up where there is high local pressure, usually between bony prominences and the shoes. Favourite areas include the upper surfaces of the toe joints and the soles just behind the toes. Soggy 'soft corns' can arise on the third or fourth toe clefts when the toes are squeezed together by shoes which are too tight.

The obvious treatment for corns is to get rid of the pressure which caused them, but many people are slow to accept this. Regular paring may make life more comfortable for a while, but only a switch to looser shoes will achieve a permanent effect. Corns under the feet can be helped by the use of spongy soft soles, but sometimes orthopaedic advice is needed to alter the pattern of weight-bearing. Particular care is needed for corns on the feet of people with diabetes or poor circulation as these can become infected or ulcerated.

SKIN CANCERS

Skin cancer is an increasingly common problem, particularly in fair-skinned people living in sunny climates. More attention to sun avoidance would reverse this trend, and publicity campaigns along this line have already been successful, for example, in Australia.

The best chance of a complete cure of any cancer, wherever it occurs in the body, comes if the diagnosis has been made early. This

THERE ARE THREE TYPES OF SKIN CANCER

- Malignant melanoma.
- Basal cell cancer (rodent ulcer).
- Squamous cell cancer.

gives an advantage to doctors dealing with skin cancers which can be seen as soon as they start. The problems remain, however, of recognising them as soon as they are seen.

It is because all three types may appear first as harmless looking lumps or areas of discoloration that you should see your doctor earlier rather than later if you are worried.

Malignant melanoma

There has been so much talk about these tumours in the media that most people know something about them. Luckily, melanomas are still uncommon, but, nevertheless, their numbers are doubling every ten years. They are more important than other types of skin cancer as they have a greater tendency to spread within the body.

For this reason it is particularly important to recognise and remove them early, before this has a chance to happen. If this can be achieved, a melanoma is easily curable.

Melanomas run in a few families whose members should be particularly careful about checking their moles and avoiding sunburn. Usually such a family history is absent, but others at risk tend to have more moles than average (though less than one-third of melanomas arise in pre-existing moles), and perhaps also fair or red hair and a tendency to freckle. They, too, should avoid excessive sun exposure.

Women get more melanomas than men, the most common site for them being the legs. Young men tend to get melanomas on their backs, and older people of both sexes are liable to develop them on their faces.

Any recently arrived or changing pigmented area has to be taken seriously. Melanomas often show different shades of brown or black – they may even be pink. Their edges tend to be rather irregular and they may be itchy and perhaps bleed easily.

Doctors often use the A,B,C,D rule to try and discriminate between benign and malignant moles: **A**symmetry, irregular **B**order, **C**olour variation and **D**iameter greater than 5 mm, should all raise suspicion that a mole needs expert attention.

There are, of course, plenty of other common and harmless conditions which share these

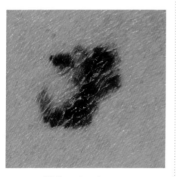

Malignant melanoma.

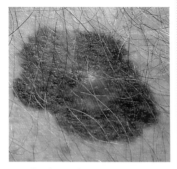
Another malignant melanoma.

features. Even so, the worst mistake is to stall and take no action for several months. You should consult your doctor early rather than late so that arrangements can be made to remove any slightly suspicious areas for checking in the laboratory.

Basal cell cancer (rodent ulcer)

This is the most common type of skin cancer and usually affects middle-aged or elderly people. Too much sun over too many years is the usual cause. These tumours grow most often on the face or neck as whitish, translucent, rather pearly lumps. After a while the centre may break down into an ulcer which bleeds and crusts from time to time. The usual story is of a small area which will not heal, but only enlarges very slowly, often taking a year or two to reach a diameter of even one centimetre.

These tumours never spread to distant parts of the body, but they do slowly enlarge locally. In doing so they can damage the nose, eye or any nearby structure. It is important that they should be treated before this can happen. They can usually be removed surgically: larger ones may need complex surgery or radiotherapy. As with all types of skin tumour, early treatment gives the best results.

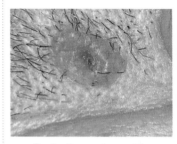
Basel cell cancer on upper lip.

Squamous cell cancer

This tumour also favours sun-damaged skin, but may even appear on skin that is usually covered. Sun is therefore not the only trigger.

A squamous cell cancer grows more quickly than a basal cell cancer. It produces an irregular, pink lump that may be quite hard and scaly, and may form an ulcer. This tumour can spread to the neighbouring lymph glands or to other parts of the body. Because of this, rapid treatment is advisable. It is usually best to remove it surgically, but radiotherapy treatment is also successful.

Birthmarks

Blemishes of various types are often seen on the skin at birth. They are made up of an incorrect mixture of the skin's usual components. For example, some birthmarks contain too many blood vessels and so look red. Others contain too much pigment and show up as brown patches or moles.

SALMON PATCHES

Small, red areas are very common on the back of the neck and, less commonly, on the forehead or upper eyelids. They are made up of dilated capillaries (the smallest blood vessels).

Those on the face usually disappear within a few months, but on the back of the neck they remain throughout life in about a quarter of the population as so-called 'stork beak marks'.

PORT WINE STAINS

Occasionally, very wide capillaries are present from birth causing a flat area of skin to be bright red or purple. This is a port wine stain. They vary in size, but a few reach several centimetres across and, unfortunately, the face is the area which is most commonly affected.

Port wine stains do not go away by themselves. They grow with the

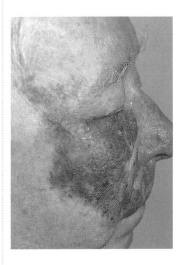

Port wine stain.

child and can be very disfiguring. Camouflage creams help a great deal and treatment with a laser is sometimes effective, although it is hard to predict who will respond best. In the last few years the tunable dye laser has become the favoured treatment in children with port wine stains.

STRAWBERRY MARKS

Strictly speaking these are not birthmarks as they appear during the first few weeks of life. They grow rapidly at the start, but reach their final size by about three months. Most remain small, but a few are several centimetres across. At their peak they are raised, soft and bright red. Thereafter, over the next four to eight years, they gradually get smaller, paler and less obvious. Most disappear without trace; some leave only a small blemish.

Bleeding can be a problem in the first year or two. This worries parents, but can be dealt with by firm pressure over the mark with a dressing or clean handkerchief. The best long-term results are obtained in most cases by simply leaving strawberry marks alone.

MOLES

Some moles are present at birth, but others appear later in childhood or adolescence. Their numbers reach a peak in early to middle

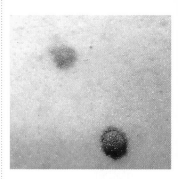

Two moles that are harmless.

adult life and then they progressively become fewer into old age. Most are small – the larger ones tend to have been present from birth. A few are very large and these are also hairy. Most people have between 15 and 20 moles.

Under the microscope moles show an abundance of melanocytes – the skin cells that produce pigment. Most moles, therefore, show up as various shades of brown though others are skin coloured. Some are flat; others are raised and shaped like a pea or a cauliflower.

The chance of an individual mole turning into a skin cancer (melanoma) is low. This is dealt with on page 35. It is sensible to see your doctor if any of your moles change, especially if they bleed, grow or alter in colour.

SKIN PIGMENT

The main pigment in our skin is melanin, and this gives the colour also to our hair and eyes. Fair-

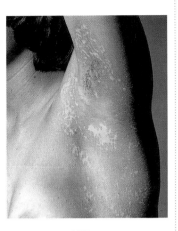

Vitiligo.

skinned people have only a little melanin – those with dark skin have a lot. The main function of melanin is to protect the skin from ultraviolet in the sun's rays. Those with very fair skin are poorly protected and so are at greater risk of sunburn and later of developing skin cancer (page 35). Albinos, who cannot make any skin pigment at all, are the most vulnerable.

The most common cause of an increase in melanin production is sun exposure. Freckles also occur where pigment cells in small areas produce too much melanin in response to sunlight. Chloasma is a darkening of the face which is usually symmetrical and like a mask.

It sometimes occurs in women who are pregnant or on the birth control pill, and is made more obvious by sun exposure. It may last for months after delivery or stopping the pill.

When the skin has been inflamed, for example, after a burn, a skin infection or even eczema, pigment may escape from pigment-producing cells in the area. This leads to a brown colour (post-inflammatory pigmentation) which may stay for some months. Paradoxically, the opposite can happen too, so that sometimes the damaged skin is left paler than before.

There are other conditions which reduce pigmentation: vitiligo is the most common of these. It affects about one in 200 of the population and occasionally is seen in more than one family member. Pigment disappears from areas of skin, usually symmetrically, leaving white areas which may increase for a few months.

Repigmentation may occur, but this is unusual and treatment tends to be ineffective. Cosmetic camouflage is often necessary if the face is affected. Sunscreens are also needed to stop the pale areas being burned.

Inherited skin conditions

In the same way as you have inherited the texture and colour of your skin and hair from your parents, so they may also have passed on to you a liability to particular skin disorders.

The three most important patterns of inheritance caused by an abnormality of only one gene are dominant, recessive and X-linked.

Dominant

These conditions pass regularly from one generation to the next, males and females being equally affected. Each child of an affected individual has a one in two chance of being affected too. Skin examples include the common minor abnormality known as 'keratosis pilaris', in which hard plugs in the hair follicles of the outer upper arms and thighs produce a rough surface, and also one common variety of dry skin (ichthyosis).

Recessive

Both parents of an affected person will be carriers of the condition, but do not show it themselves. Nevertheless, one in four of the children of a pair of carrier parents will develop the condition. Examples of this include albinism and some types of very stretchy skin.

X-linked

These show up only in males, and are carried and passed on by apparently unaffected females. The conditions therefore skip a generation and pass from grandfather to grandson. The best known example of all is haemophilia and, in the context of skin disorders, one variety of dry skin (ichthyosis).

Many other common conditions, such as psoriasis and eczema, often run in families, but in ways that do not fit with the dominant, recessive or X-linked types of inheritance. This puzzle has not yet been solved, but it seems likely that they result from abnormalities of several genes, not just of one.

The hair and nails

For many people, the hair and nails only merit attention when they need cutting. Unlike skin, which grows continuously outwards, each hair grows for a few months but then goes into a resting phase and is later shed. In contrast, nails continue to grow out along the nail bed and, if left uncut, will finally break from some minor injury. If looked after carefully, nails will grow up to one foot in length.

The cosmetic importance of hair and nails cannot be overestimated. Advertisements always feature people with sleek, thick hair and perfect, pink, well-groomed nails. This public image of 'nice' hair inculcates ideas about its colour, thickness, manageability and growth pattern. With nails, function is more important than appearance. The ability to pick up small items is crucial in many occupations and in everyday life. In this chapter we deal with some diseases which can seriously affect the appearance of hair and nails or interfere with their function. We also mention some which may alert a doctor to other problems.

HAIR

Too little hair

● **Common baldness:** some degree of common (androgenic) baldness is normal in men and women from puberty onwards. Most men have to accept that their hairline will recede and that they may go a bit thin on top, too. Sons may follow a family pattern in this respect, and hair loss may become quite noticeable by the age of 30. Fortunately, most women keep good heads of hair right into old age. Some slight thinning is inevitable, but a few women, even in their 30s, may also get thin on top.

We know that most of them have normal hormone concentrations, but that their hair roots are oversensitive even to these normal levels. Thinning is especially embarrassing for women, and if their problem is severe some feel the need to wear a wig. To come to terms with baldness, a full explanation is needed. If trying to cope causes major emotional problems, the individual is often found to have been prone to emotional problems anyway. Thin hair is upsetting, but it is not the end of the world and most people adjust successfully to it.

Cyproterone acetate can be a useful treatment for women. It is an anti-androgen and is used in combination with an oestrogen in the pill Dianette. It may help acne, androgenic baldness and excess hair on the rest of the body. However, the improvement is rarely dramatic and lasts only as long as treatment is continued – and of course the usual complications of the pill must be considered. Both men and women can try a lotion containing minoxidil, but, again, there are problems. The lotion is expensive and not available on the NHS. It has to be applied indefinitely and, even then, the effects are often disappointing. Indeed, in most people, little or no effect can be seen.

Surgery is another approach, but is perhaps a little drastic. Three techniques can be used. The first is to remove 3 mm cylindrical pieces of hair-bearing skin from the back of the scalp; these are then transplanted to the bald area where similar pieces of skin have already been removed. This is like planting little pots of seedlings in rows. In the second technique a central bald patch is cut out from the crown and the edges are sewn together. Finally, there is a difficult technique in which a flap of hair-bearing skin is moved forwards to cover a bald area without interrupting its blood supply.

• **Alopecia areata:** this is the medical term for loss of hair in patches. It may occasionally cause a more widespread hair loss and, rarely, every hair may be lost from the body. The cause is unknown, but the condition may run in families.

It usually starts in childhood or early adult life. The bald patches usually regrow, but new ones may continue to appear. Sadly, in a few people, there is little regrowth. Doctors may recommend creams, ultraviolet light or injection into the bald areas, but although these measures can sometimes speed up the process of regrowth, they do not, unfortunately, prevent further patches developing. Occasionally, only the pigmented hair falls out leaving any grey ones untouched. When this happens people suddenly seem to go grey overnight.

- **Traction:** when hair is pulled hard its roots may come out. Certain hairstyles put extra stress on the hair and may pull out enough to cause thinning. Ponytails are one example, as is the tight plaiting of the hair.
- **Telogen effluvium:** during pregnancy the hair often looks particularly thick; the price may be paid a few months later when all the hairs which have been growing in unison are shed at the same time. This is called telogen effluvium and the result can be noticeable hair loss. It is of course followed by regrowth.

This process may also be seen a few months after any acute and severe illness.
- **Chronic widespread alopecia:** hair may be lost evenly over the entire scalp in association with various general diseases. It then regrows when the underlying disease is sorted out. Examples of these illnesses are thyroid disease, iron deficiency, malabsorption, plus some medications, including warfarin.
- **Scarring alopecia:** if the hair follicles are destroyed, obviously new hairs cannot reappear, and the baldness is therefore irreversible. Some examples of this situation are physical injuries (e.g. burns), severe fungal infections, bacterial infections and some skin diseases, e.g. lichen planus and lupus erythematosus.

Too much hair

Men grow coarse hairs over wider areas than women. Hirsutism is the term for the growth of hair in women in a typically male pattern. Many women develop a slight increase in hair on the face, around the nipples and in other areas, but this is seldom the result of any disease. It occurs for reasons similar to those that cause baldness in men and thinning of scalp hair in women – that is, the hair roots are over-reacting to normal hormone concentrations in the blood.

The contraceptive pill may delay the changes and some women notice a slight increase in face or body hair within two years of stopping the pill. When a woman seeks advice about excess hair her doctor must try to assess how real the problem is. In the West there is a media-driven obsession with hair. The 'normal' woman is portrayed as having no hair except on the scalp, but in reality many women do have some body hair. This tendency runs in families and is more common in some racial groups, e.g. in Mediterranean types. The second point is that some people who complain of excessive hairiness have, in fact, only an abnormal perception of themselves and appear quite normal to other people. Third, the doctor has to decide if the excess hair is due to an underlying disease or medication.

Many women who dislike their excess hair also dislike the idea of prolonged treatment. Depilatory creams may help, though in some they cause soreness. Waxing and shaving are other purely temporary measures. Electrolysis is a permanent method, but each hair may have to be treated two or three times, making it time-consuming and expensive. What happens is that the therapist places a fine needle down the side of each hair shaft before activating an electric current. In good hands this leaves little or no scaring, but overactive or clumsy treatment can leave some dimpling. The hormone cyproterone acetate can help, but is only a temporary measure and hair reappears if the drug is stopped. Hair clinics offer many different treatments, but we have seen no evidence that they work well.

NAILS

Fingernails grow at the rate of about 1 cm in three months and toe nails at abut 1 cm in six months. This explains why it takes so long for a damaged or diseased nail to grow out. The visible part of the nail is hard and inert – it can be injured or infected by fungus, but little else can happen to it. The growing part of the nail (nail matrix) lies beneath and behind the cuticle and also forms the half moons which are usually visible. Disease of the matrix produces certain characteristic changes such as thin, thick, pitted or rough nails.

Ingrowing toe nails

These are often a great nuisance. Uncommon before 10 and after 25, they are partly caused by poorly fitting shoes. They do not occur in the barefoot and were especially common in those who wore winklepicker shoes. The big toe nail digs into the skin on either side, making it sore and easily infected. Helpful measures include cutting the nail straight across, wearing loose shoes and putting a small wad of cotton wool under the nail

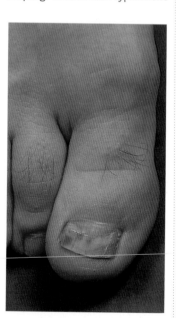

Fungus damage to nails.

corners. Sometimes it is necessary to remove a strip of nail at the edge to allow the skin to heal.

Infection

If an infection develops under the cuticle (paronychia), pain and swelling are inevitable and pus may seep out. The best treatment is then with antibiotics. Sudden or acute infections may come out of the blue, but more commonly they occur in people with chronically damaged cuticles.

Anyone engaged regularly in wet work, e.g. hairdressing or washing, is at risk, and the skin surrounding the nail may become permanently red, swollen and tender. To clear this up the hands should be kept warm and dry cotton gloves should be worn inside rubber gloves at work. Sometimes yeasts get into the damaged areas and appropriate creams can then give relief. Herpes virus may also infect a finger, causing a herpetic whitlow. Swelling and pain with little blisters may last for a week or so.

Some fungi can infect the nails and usually do so in association with another focus of infection, for example, in athletes' foot between the toes. The great toenails are most often affected. There may simply be a whitening of the nail surface or a whole nail may become thickened, crumbly and yellow. It is not necessary to treat most fungal toenail infections, but help is needed if the finger nails are involved. Once the diagnosis has been confirmed, anti-fungal tablets must be taken for weeks or months. Newer drugs are more effective, but there is still a high recurrence rate within a year of stopping therapy.

Brittle nails

Some nails split easily, either by peeling of very thin layers at the free edge or by splitting longitudinally. Housewives are particularly prone to these problems as they repeatedly wet their hands. Some varnishes damage the top layer, as indeed do some varnish removers. The best remedy is to wear light cotton inners under rubber gloves when in contact with water. Minerals and vitamin supplements are rarely helpful.

Thick, hard nails

Huge, thick yellowish nails may slowly appear in some elderly people. Occasionally a curly horn-like shape emerges. Such nails are impossible to cut and even chiropodists have difficulty with them. Older people may find they cannot reach their toenails to cut them, or that poor eyesight makes it hazardous to try. Repeated damage to the nail over a lifetime, coupled with poor circulation, both contribute to this condition.

Other disease and the nails

Some skin diseases are accompanied by changes in the nails. In psoriasis the nail surface may be pitted like a thimble or the nails may thicken or even lift off the nail-bed, allowing air and dirt to get underneath.

Eczema often causes irregular dents and roughening of the surface.

Internal diseases occasionally produce nail changes too. Iron deficiency leads to flat or spooned nails, and liver disease may produce white nails.

Sunlight and its effects

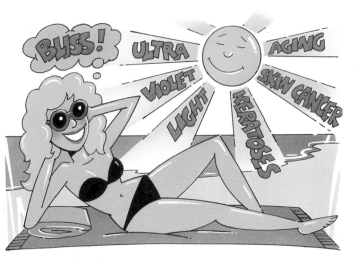

Natural sunlight is made up of heat, visible light and ultraviolet light. These are mainly beneficial to humans, but when problems do arise they are caused by the ultraviolet component.

Ultraviolet light itself is divided into three types – A, B and C, usually referred to as UV-A, and UV-B and UV-C. Worries over thinning of the ozone layer centre upon the possibility that more UV-B and UV-C will get through the atmosphere to damage our skin. To understand the role of sunlight in our lives we have to think both about its benefits and its harmful effects.

BENEFITS

Some vitamin D, which is essential for a healthy life, is made in skin exposed to sunlight: lack of vitamin D eventually leads to rickets. Also, those who have been exposed to sunlight often say that they feel particularly well. It is impossible to measure these feelings scientifically, but the existence of such a benefit cannot be ignored.

In addition, dermatologists often use UV-A and UV-B to treat skin diseases. Not all will respond, but two which tend to do well are acne and psoriasis.

HARMFUL EFFECTS

We are all familiar with lobster-coloured sunbathers who have badly estimated the sun's intensity. Fair-skinned people learn the hard way at an early age that they must avoid prolonged sun exposure: their skin contains little melanin, the protective pigment, whereas darker and black skins have much larger amounts. Current thinking is that young skin is particularly susceptible to ultraviolet light and the damage done is irreversible. Children must be protected and sunburn at this age is a parental responsibility. Severe sunburn is painful, and obviously should be avoided, but there are also less evident, long-term dangers associated with too much sun exposure. These can be separated into four groups.

Solar keratoses

These are rough, scaly, sun-induced patches occurring on the head, neck or backs of hands. Bald people may get them on their scalp. Their bases are red and on top they are rough, like sandpaper, or crusted.

It is total exposure to sunlight over a lifetime that is important here, and anyone who has spent a long time in the sun, even 20 years ago, is liable to develop solar keratoses. The same rule, incidentally, also applies to the development of flat, brown patches (liver spots or lentigos).

Most solar keratoses remain benign, and can be treated easily by freezing them with liquid nitrogen. A very few may eventually turn into squamous cell cancer (page 36).

Skin cancers

Each of the three most common skin cancers (page 34) appears most often in those who have had too much sun exposure. The sun can do its damage at any age, but the growths do not usually appear until middle or old age. Ultraviolet light is not the only cause of skin cancer, but large doses of it increase the chance of one developing.

Ageing

Another long-term hazard of sunlight (mainly its UV-A component) is ageing of the skin. The bronzed, young skins of today

DOS AND DON'TS

Always avoid getting burned by the sun, and this must include avoiding the sun when it is at its height for three hours around midday. A slight tan may be safe, but it is not a good idea to sunbathe solidly for a fortnight every year or to keep your tan going artificially. Remember that sunscreens are not a substitute for sun avoidance and sensible protective clothing. They do not protect the skin from all components of the sun's rays: indeed, those that mainly block UV-B may lessen the chance of acute sunburn, but in doing so allow you to spend more time in the sun and so get an excessive dose of ageing UV-A rays.

Nevertheless, sunscreens blocking both UV-A and UV-B are still useful. Sun protection factors (SPF) are marked on most products and indicate how much longer than usual an individual will be able to stay in the sun. In other words, if you can expect to tolerate 5 minutes on day 1 of your holiday without protection, then SPF 10 products will allow you to stay out for 50 minutes. They do wash and rub off, so apply more cream from time to time and always after swimming; and remember that sun will also penetrate thin clothes.

Sunbeds and sunlamps in sun parlours or at home are, we hope, a declining industry nowadays. These machines give out unpredictable mixtures of wavelengths, including UV-A and UV-B. After all that has been said in this section, it should be clear why doctors never encourage people to use them without medical supervision. Certainly they should never be used just for a spurious sense of 'well-being'.

The question sometimes arises as to whether someone with a chronic skin disease should have a lamp at home to avoid repeated, time-consuming visits to hospital. There are no easy rules here and it is best to discuss this with your own doctor.

will become the wrinkled, prune-like ones of tomorrow. You need to look no further than the leathery faces of many Mediterranean men and women to realise that it is not only the fair-skinned who are at risk. Irreversible wrinkling and loss of elasticity is the price which eventually has to be paid for the so-called 'healthy' tan that everyone has been so keen to achieve until quite recently.

Sun sensitivity

In a few people, sunlight may be the sole cause of distressing rashes on exposed areas of skin. These may be difficult to control and even minute amounts of ultraviolet light can keep them from going out in the light. Certain medicines, for example, water tablets (diuretics) or antibiotics, can bring on this type of sun sensitivity. Other chemicals and drugs act in the same way when put directly on to the skin: chemicals in some shampoos or perfumes may be culprits here, and sunlight sets off the reaction only in areas of contact.

Surgery

The word 'surgery' has always conjured up the idea of cutting out diseased tissues from the body. In recent years it has gained a broader meaning: not only is cutting no longer a requirement, for example, laser surgery may not cut the skin, but also cosmetic surgery is performed on perfectly healthy tissue.

In addition to cosmetic surgery (to improve appearance by reversing the effects of age or altering the shapes of noses, ears, etc.), we now also use the word surgery to cover the destruction of cells by cold (cryosurgery) and the destruction of tissue with narrow wavebands of light (laser surgery).

BIOPSIES

A small piece of skin can be removed, using a scalpel, and sent to the laboratory for processing and viewing under a microscope to give a diagnosis. This is a diagnostic biopsy, a common procedure in dermatology units. The tissue normally comes from a rash or a tumour. The biopsy is normally 1 to 2 cm long and 0.3 to 0.5 cm wide. The full thickness of skin is taken, but if the disease is thought to go deeper, the biopsy must also include fat below the skin. The wound will be sewn up using two or three stitches. The results are normally available within one week.

EXCISIONAL SURGERY

When a skin lump, mole or cancer has to be removed, the technique is called excision. Essentially this is the same as a biopsy, but the entire lesion must be taken away. If there is any concern about malignancy, then a rim of healthy skin must be removed as well. Local anaesthetic is first injected under the lump, then the piece of skin is cut out and the wound is sewn up with a few stitches.

CURETTAGE

Several benign skin tumours grow from the top layer of the skin. After injecting local anaesthetic, a sharp, spoon-like instrument can be used to scoop them off the surface – a cleavage plane opens up and there is little bleeding. The scar heals well or virtually disappears as the scraping is so superficial. Viral warts, seborrhoeic warts and molluscum contagiosum can be treated in this way.

CRYOSURGERY

This is the use of cold temperatures to destroy living cells. Liquid nitrogen has a temperature of $-196°C$ and is the most effective agent. Freezing tissues to very low temperatures damages the cells, partly by the formation of ice crystals but it also leads to swelling and bursting of cells. Viral warts, solar keratoses and small seborrhoeic warts respond well to cryotherapy. The liquid can be applied with either a cotton-wool swab or a pressurised spray.

PLASTIC SURGERY

Once the decision has been made to remove a lump the surgeon must judge whether it will be possible to cut it out and join up the edges directly or whether a skin graft will be required to fill the gap. The skilful repair of skin, whether for tumour removal, burns or major abnormalities, has come to be known as plastic surgery. Skilled surgeons, whether dermatologists or plastic surgeons, need to know how skin differs from one person to another, that different areas vary in thickness and colour, and also about the way that the skin changes with age. These factors must be taken into consideration when deciding on the best operation for each individual.

Skin grafting is the removal of skin from one area to cover another. It may involve the full thickness of the skin or only part of it. Both donor and recipient areas must be matched for colour and hairiness. If for example, eyebrow skin has been removed it is better to replace it with skin from the scalp than with non-hairy skin from the thigh.

Skin flaps are commonly used to repair large defects after tumour removal. The principle is that, in tight skin areas, e.g. the nose wound closure is easier if looser skin from the cheek or forehead can be borrowed. The 'borrowed' skin is not severed completely from its surroundings, as in a skin graft, but is released on two or three sides and underneath so that it can then be stretched or slid sideways to help fit the defect.

COSMETIC SURGERY

Cosmetic surgery has become popular recently, both with patients and with some doctors. Few of us think that we look perfect, but most of us are not keen to improve our looks by subjecting ourselves to surgery.

Whether a skin blemish can be removed on the NHS depends on just how unsightly it is, and on the funds available to your local dermatologist or plastic surgeon, as this type of 'cosmetic' work has a low priority.

Plastic surgeons outside the NHS may be asked to reverse the ravages of time, such as wrinkles, crow's feet and sagging skin. However, a face lift simply tightens the skin on the face – it does not make it young again. To get an idea of how a face lift would affect your appearance, you should look into a mirror and gently pull the skin from your cheek to your ear, and from the forehead to your hairline. Having established that it will make things look better, the surgeon then cuts around the hairline and in front of the ears, frees the skin over the cheeks, gently tightens it and removes redundant skin before sewing the area together again.

LASER SURGERY

This type of surgery now overlaps with all the other types we have mentioned because different lasers have different properties.

A carbon dioxide laser is used as a light scalpel, cutting the skin accurately and sealing the blood vessels as it goes. It can, therefore, be used for malignant tumours or simply for an unsightly mole.

Other lasers have been designed specifically for purple birthmarks and can give good results. Yet another laser has been developed to treat tattoos, but this is classed as cosmetic. Better lasers will surely be developed, and will lead to improvements in the treatment of a wide variety of diseases.

Leg ulcers

These have always been a huge problem. At any time there are some 200,000 people with leg ulcers in Britain. Most are women aged over 60. Caring for them takes up to 10 per cent of a district nurse's working time.

Ulcers appear for many reasons, which have varied over the years. In the past, malnutrition or infections e.g. tuberculosis and syphilis, were often to blame. Nowadays abnormalities of the veins and arteries are usually responsible. Several causes often work together to trigger a breakdown of skin on the lower leg. Later other factors may come into play to delay healing. Most commonly there is an underlying disorder of the veins, which may be congenital or follow a thrombosis.

In some occupations prolonged standing is an extra problem. Other contributory causes include cuts, dermatitis, excessive weight, diabetes and diseases of the arteries.

It follows that there is no universal treatment for ulcers. This must depend on the cause, and should be tailored to each patient. Ulcers resulting from diabetes or arterial disease need a different approach which may involve taking an X-ray of the blood vessels supplying the leg (an arteriogram). Ulcers thought to result from disease of the veins are investigated by taking the blood pressure in the foot and in the arm, and comparing the two. If the pressure in the foot is almost as high as in the arm, the arteries are working well, and it will be safe to apply compression bandages to the leg. These are wrapped around the foot, ankle and up the leg at the correct tension and left on for several days at a time. They compress the veins in the skin and encourage blood to flow up large veins deeper in the calf. Compression bandages are perhaps the most important part of treatment, but are not the whole story and not always easy to tolerate. Some people have painful or weeping ulcers, odd shaped legs, and other problems which make compression unsuitable.

Ulcers must be cleaned, but they are open wounds and bound to have bacteria growing on their surfaces. Small ones respond to a variety of gentle, moist dressings. Antiseptics are sometimes used. The surrounding skin should be moisturised or treated with a weak steroid cream if there are signs of eczema. The dressing is covered by a retaining bandage, followed by a soft material, such as wool felt, and the compression bandage then goes on top.

As an ulcer improves, a change from compression bandages to compression stockings may be possible. These can be made to measure but are still quite difficult to put on, especially for those who find it difficult to bend or who have a weak grip due to arthritis.

Keeping an ulcer healed is often as difficult as healing it in the first place. General measures which are also of use in the healing phase include weight reduction, keeping mobile, concentrating on ankle movements, and a slight elevation of the foot of the bed at night.

Other associated conditions

OTHER DISEASES

Most of the conditions in this book have their main impact on the skin, where they cause itching, discomfort, embarrassment, etc. However, other diseases have their main effects internally and only affect the skin to a lesser degree. Even so, sometimes these skin changes help doctors to identify an underlying disorder.

For example, diabetes may show up as a tendency to get thrush, or by the appearance on the shins of shiny yellow–red areas known as necrobiosis. An overactive thyroid gland can lead to sweating and an underactive one to dry itchy skin; both may cause hair loss. An excess of lipids (fat) in the blood can be deposited in the skin as yellow patches or lumps.

Malnutrition may lead to a scaly, itchy skin, with changes in pigmentation. Problems are also seen in other deficiency states, e.g.

lack of vitamin C causes scurvy and bruising; lack of iron causes sores at the corners of the mouth with general itching. A smooth tongue may be seen in iron deficiency, pernicious anaemia (vitamin B_{12} deficiency) and when food is not absorbed properly.

Occasionally internal cancers affect the skin, and doctors are on the look out for these changes, which are rare and beyond the scope of this book. Nevertheless, they act as a reminder that the skin can mirror problems in any other organ. Finally, some drugs have side effects and the skin is one site in which these can show up. Several patterns may be seen as shown in the table on page 57.

THE SKIN AND STRESS

It is wrong to assume, as so many do, that stress is important in every skin condition – but sometimes undoubtedly it is. The process

PATTERNS SHOWN AS DRUG SIDE EFFECTS

Type of eruption	Example of drug	Used for
Blisters	Frusemide	Heart failure, swollen legs
	Penicillamine	Rheumatoid arthritis
Red skin all over	Allopurinol	Gout
	Phenytoin	Epilepsy
Excessive sensitivity to light	Chlorpropamide	Diabetes
Pigmentation	Minocycline	Acne
Urticaria	Aspirin	Aches and pains
	Penicillin	Infections
Like psoriasis	Beta blockers	Angina, blood pressure

works in both directions. People can react to a skin condition by becoming excessively worried about it; in contrast, stress can worsen or even trigger some skin problems.

In areas such as the face, scalp and genitals, even very minor skin changes can lead to much anxiety and loss of self-esteem. An extreme form of this is when people become depressed about things that no-one else even notices. A few people also cling on to mistaken beliefs about their skin, sometimes believing, for example, that it is infested with parasites despite evidence to the contrary.

Nervous tension itself can lead to a variety of minor habits, such as picking and digging at the skin, or at acne spots. Some people rub at itchy areas of skin until they become thickened and discoloured (neurodermatitis). Some children bite their nails, or pull and twist their hair while doing their homework. Often it is best not to protest too strongly, as this can perpetuate habits which otherwise would have gone away by themselves.

Other skin conditions which are triggered or worsened by stress include psoriasis, urticaria, eczema and alopecia areata. Fancy rather than fact rules here, and proof is often lacking. Unfortunately the use of tranquillisers or psychiatric treatment seldom seems to help very much.

Useful Addresses

ACNE
Acne Support Group
PO Box 230, Hayes
Middlesex UB4 9HW

ALLERGY
British Allergy Foundation
c/o Professor Robert Davies
St Bartholomew's Hospital
West Smithfield, London EC1A 7BE

COSMETIC COVER
British Red Cross Society
COSCAM Beauty Care Development
9 Grosvenor Crescent, London SW1X 7EJ

ECZEMA
National Eczema Society
163 Eversholt Street
London NW1 1BU

HAIR
Alopecia Patients' Society
39 St John's Close
Knowle, Solihull
B93 0NN

HERPES
Herpes Association
c/o Mr Michael Wolfe
41 North Road, London N7 9DP

LUPUS
Lupus UK
c/o B. Hanner
51 North Street, Romford, Essex RM1 1BA

MELANOMA
Melanoma Network
c/o Mr John Tresidder
23 Fairways Road, Seaford, Sussex BN2 54E

NAEVI
Naevus Support Group
58 Necton Road, Wheathampstead
Hertfordshire AL4 8AU

PSORIASIS
The Psoriasis Association
Milton House, 7 Milton Street
Northampton NN2 7JG

The Psoriatic Arthropathy Support Group
c/o Mr David Chandler, 136 High Street
Bushey, Hertfordshire WD2 3DJ

SCLERODERMA
The Scleroderma Society
c/o Mrs P. Webster, 61 Sandpit Lane
St Albans, Hertfordshire AL1 4EY

VITILIGO
The Vitiligo Society
19 Fitzroy Square, London W1P 5HQ

Index